WATSU AQUATIC THERAPY

A Guide to Water-Based Healing for Mind, Body, and Spirit: Fundamentals to Advanced Practices, Customized Sessions, Rehabilitation Strategies, Mental Wellness Applications

WILFREDO CARSON

Watsu Aquatic Therapy: With Expert Guidance" is a pioneering manual that delves deep into the transformative potential of aquatic therapy, offering a comprehensive roadmap for both beginners and seasoned practitioners.

At its core, this book reveals the profound principles of Watsu, an innovative therapeutic approach that harnesses the power of water to heal and rejuvenate the mind and body. Through meticulous exploration, readers embark on a journey through the rich history and evolution of aquatic therapy, gaining insights into its myriad benefits for holistic wellness.

From improving physical mobility to fostering emotional resilience, Watsu emerges as a versatile modality capable of addressing a wide range of health concerns.

Each chapter is a treasure trove of knowledge, offering practical advice, step-by-step instructions, and insightful anecdotes to enrich the learning experience.

These pages guide readers through every aspect of Watsu practice, from creating a safe and nurturing aquatic environment to mastering advanced techniques for deep tissue release and energy balancing. One of the book's most compelling features is its emphasis on customization and adaptability.

Whether tailoring sessions to meet individual needs or adapting techniques for diverse populations, Watsu's flexibility shines through as a modality that can be tailored to a variety of contexts and preferences. Furthermore, "Watsu Aquatic Therapy" demonstrates the profound intersection of physical rehabilitation and mental wellness. Through real-life case studies and expert insights, readers gain a deeper understanding of how Watsu can be used not only to address physical ailments, but also to promote emotional healing and psychological well-being.

As readers progress through the pages of this book, they are not only given the tools and techniques they need to excel in their practice, but also inspired to imagine the limitless possibilities that lie ahead.

From forging meaningful connections within healthcare communities to embracing cutting-edge innovations in aquatic therapy technology, the future of Watsu is illuminated as a beacon of hope and healing for generations to come.

CHAPTER 1
INTRODUCTION TO WATSU AQUATIC THERAPY

Watsu Aquatic Therapy is an aquatic bodywork modality that combines shiatsu massage and water-based movements to promote relaxation, healing, and overall well-being. Developed in the 1980s by Harold Dull, Watsu has gained recognition for its unique approach to healing in water. This therapeutic practice involves gentle stretching, rhythmic movements, and pressure point manipulation in a warm pool. The buoyancy Understanding the principles of watsu: At the core of Watsu Aquatic Therapy lie several principles that guide its practice and effectiveness.

Central to these principles is the concept of water as a medium for healing and transformation.

Water's buoyancy reduces the effects of gravity, relieving pressure on joints and allowing for fluid movements that may be difficult to achieve on land. Additionally, the warmth of the water promotes muscle relaxation and increases circulation, facilitating the release of tension and promoting overall relaxation.

Another key principle of Watsu is the integration of shiatsu techniques, which involve applying pressure to specific points along the body's meridians to stimulate energy flow and promote balance. By combining these techniques with the fluidity of water, Watsu practitioners can create a deeply therapeutic experience that addresses both physical and energetic imbalances. Furthermore, Watsu emphasizes the importance of connection and trust between practitioner and client, fostering a supportive environment conducive to healing and personal growth. Through the application of these principles, Watsu Aquatic Therapy offers a unique and effective approach to holistic wellness.

History and Development of Aquatic Therapy:

The history of aquatic therapy dates back centuries, with cultures around the world recognizing the healing properties of water. Ancient civilizations, such as the Greeks and Romans, utilized hydrotherapy for its therapeutic benefits, including pain relief, relaxation, and rejuvenation. However, the modern practice of aquatic therapy, including Watsu, has its roots in the latter half of the 20th century.

Harold Dull, a massage therapist and aquatic bodywork pioneer, is credited with developing Watsu in the early 1980s. Drawing inspiration from techniques he learned in Japan, Dull began exploring the potential of water as a medium for healing and self-discovery.

Over time, he refined his approach, combining elements of shiatsu massage, yoga, and meditation to create the practice now known as Watsu. Since its inception, Watsu has continued to evolve, with practitioners incorporating new techniques and insights to enhance its effectiveness. Today, Watsu is practiced worldwide and has gained recognition for its profound therapeutic benefits across diverse populations, including individuals with physical disabilities, chronic pain, and mental health concerns. As the field of aquatic therapy continues to grow, so too does our understanding of its history, evolution, and potential for promoting health and well-being. Watsu benefits the mind and body. The benefits of Watsu Aquatic Therapy are wide-ranging and encompass both physical and mental aspects of wellness.

One of the primary advantages of Watsu is its ability to promote relaxation and reduce stress. The warm water and gentle movements of Watsu induce a state of deep relaxation, helping to calm the nervous system and alleviate tension held in the body.

This relaxation response can have numerous positive effects, including reduced muscle pain, improved sleep quality, and enhanced mood. Additionally, Watsu can be beneficial for improving flexibility and range of motion, particularly for individuals with musculoskeletal conditions or mobility limitations. The buoyancy of water supports the body, allowing for gentle stretching and movement without putting strain on the joints. For individuals recovering from injury or surgery, Watsu can also aid in rehabilitation by promoting circulation, reducing inflammation, and facilitating the healing process. Beyond its physical benefits, Watsu has been shown to have profound effects on mental well-being. The combination of water's soothing properties and the nurturing touch of the practitioner creates a safe and supportive environment for emotional release and healing.

Many clients report feelings of deep peace, connection, and inner harmony after a Watsu session, which can have lasting effects on their overall sense of well-being. Moreover, Watsu has been found to be particularly effective for managing symptoms of anxiety, depression, and trauma-related stress, offering a gentle yet powerful approach to mental health support. Overall, the holistic nature of Watsu Aquatic Therapy makes it a valuable tool for promoting health and healing on multiple levels, making it an essential component of comprehensive wellness care.

CHAPTER 2
GETTING STARTED WITH WATSU

Watsu, an abbreviation for "Water Shiatsu," is a unique form of aquatic bodywork that combines elements of massage, stretching, and joint mobilization in a warm water environment. It is characterized by its gentle, fluid movements and supportive buoyancy, which provide a profound sense of relaxation and release. Getting started with Watsu requires understanding its principles, techniques, and benefits, as well as the necessary preparations and precautions to ensure a safe and Preparing for Watsu Practice. To practice Watsu, you must first prepare yourself physically, mentally, and emotionally. This includes cultivating a

pg. 16

mindset of mindfulness, compassion, and presence, as well as ensuring that you are physically fit and capable of performing the necessary movements and techniques. Maintaining proper hygiene, such as showering before entering the water and wearing appropriate swimwear, is also crucial to uphold professional standards. Setting up the aquatic environment. Creating an optimal aquatic environment is essential for the practice of Watsu, as it influences the overall experience and outcomes of the session. The water temperature should be comfortably warm, typically between 92°F and 98°F, to promote relaxation and muscle release while preventing discomfort or hypothermia. The pool or body of water should be clean and free of debris, with adequate depth to allow for fluid movement and buoyancy.

Furthermore, providing supportive Safety Concerns and Precautions Safety is paramount in Watsu practice, as working in the water presents unique risks and challenges that must be addressed to ensure the well-being of both the practitioner and the client. Practitioners should be trained in water safety, CPR, and rescue techniques to respond effectively to emergencies and mitigate potential hazards. Prior to each session, a thorough assessment of the client's medical history, physical condition, and any contraindications to aquatic therapy should be conducted to tailor the session accordingly and avoid exacerbating existing injuries or conditions. Furthermore, maintaining clear communication and boundaries with the client throughout the session is essential to ensure their comfort, consent, and autonomy.

Regular maintenance and inspection of equipment, facilities, and water quality are also crucial to prevent accidents or contamination.

By adhering to these safety considerations and precautions, practitioners can create a secure and supportive environment for the practice of Watsu, facilitating optimal outcomes and client satisfaction.

CHAPTER 3
BASIC TECHNIQUES IN WATSU

Watsu, a type of aquatic bodywork therapy, encompasses various fundamental techniques aimed at promoting relaxation, healing, and overall well-being.

These techniques leverage the unique properties of water to facilitate physical and mental benefits for individuals seeking therapeutic interventions. Watsu is a therapy that focuses on conscious breathing to deepen relaxation and improve the mind-body connection.

By focusing on the breath, individuals can cultivate a state of mindfulness and presence, allowing them to release tension and quiet the chatter of their minds.

Practitioners guide clients in sy Moreover, Watsu incorporates gentle movement and stretching sequences designed to promote flexibility, mobility, and release of muscular tension. These sequences are tailored to meet the unique needs and abilities of each individual, ensuring a personalized approach to therapeutic intervention.

By gently manipulating the body in water, practitioners can facilitate greater freedom of movement without the constraints imposed by gravity. Participants experience a sense of weightlessness and ease as they engage in fluid movements that promote circulation, joint mobility, and overall vitality. The warm, supportive environment of the water enhances the effectiveness of these movements, allowing individuals to experience a deeper level of relaxation and release.

Through regular practice of gentle movement and stretching sequences, clients can experience improvements in range of motion, posture, and overall physical well-being, contributing to their overall quality of life and sense of vitality.

CHAPTER 4
ADVANCED WATSU TECHNIQUES

Advanced Watsu techniques encompass a range of specialized practices that go beyond the fundamental principles of water-based therapy. These techniques are designed to offer deeper levels of healing and relaxation to individuals seeking alternative forms of treatment for various physical and psychological conditions. Deep tissue release and joint mobilization, for example, involves targeted manipulation of soft tissues and joints within the aquatic environment. Shiatsu massage, which originated in Japan, is a form of bodywork that involves applying rhythmic pressure to specific points along the body's meridians to promote energy flow and restore balance. When applied to the aquatic setting, Shiatsu techniques can enhance the therapeutic effects of Watsu by stimulating acupressure points and facilitating the release of tension and stress. In Watsu, therapists can manipulate the flow of water and guide clients through fluid movements to influence the subtle energy currents within the body, promoting Advanced Watsu techniques offer a multifaceted approach to water-based healing, integrating elements of massage therapy, energy work, and aquatic movement to address the diverse needs of clients. Through deep tissue release and joint mobilization, therapists can target specific areas of tension and dysfunction, promoting physical rehabilitation and pain relief. Shiatsu massage principles can be used to enhance the therapeutic effects of Watsu by harm.

CHAPTER 5
CUSTOMIZING WATU SESSIONS

Customizing Watsu sessions, which are based on the principles of aquatic bodywork and Shiatsu massage, is a critical part of ensuring that individuals seeking water-based healing get the most out of the therapy. By addressing specific physical, emotional, and mental concerns, practitioners can improve the therapy's overall effectiveness. Sessions are tailored to individual needs. To tailor Watsu sessions to individual needs, the practitioner must first conduct a thorough consultation to gather relevant information about the client's medical history, current physical condition, and any specific areas of concern. By understanding the client's unique needs, the practitioner can design a personalized treatment plan that aligns Adapting Watsu to Different Populations: Adapting Watsu for different populations is essential for ensuring inclusivity and accessibility within the realm of aquatic therapy. Various demographic groups, such as seniors, athletes, and pregnant individuals, may have distinct physiological and psychological needs that necessitate tailored approaches to Watsu. For seniors, gentle movements and buoyancy support can help alleviate joint stiffness and improve mobility, enhancing overall quality of life. Athletes, on the

Integrating Music, Aromatherapy, and Other Enhancements

Music, known for its ability to evoke emotions and induce relaxation, can complement the rhythmic movements of Watsu, fostering a harmonious connection between mind and body. By choosing appropriate musical compositions, practitioners can create an immersive environment conducive to stress reduction and emotional release. In conclusion, customizing Watsu sessions entails tailoring the therapy to individual needs, adapting it for different populations, and incorporating complementary enhancements such as music and aromatherapy. By adopting these concepts, practitioners can optimize the therapeutic outcomes of Watsu, fostering holistic healing for the mind, body, and spirit. Watsu emerges as a versatile modality through personalized approaches and thoughtful integration of sensory elements.

CHAPTER 6
WATSU FOR REHABILITATION AND HEALING

Watsu, a type of aquatic therapy, has gained attention for its potential to promote rehabilitation and healing across a wide range of conditions. This modality harnesses the therapeutic properties of water to facilitate physical, emotional, and mental well-being. Within the realm of rehabilitation and healing, Watsu offers a holistic approach that integrates movement, buoyancy, and mindful presence to address specific conditions and foster recovery.

Addressing specific conditions: Watsu therapy can be tailored to address a wide range of specific conditions, including chronic pain, post-surgery recovery, and posttraumatic stress disorder (PTSD). In the context of chronic pain management, Watsu's gentle movements and warm water environment can provide relief by promoting muscle relaxation, increasing circulation, and releasing endorphins, which act as natural pain relievers. Watsu also offers a low-impact Case Studies, Success Stories: Numerous case studies and success stories attest to the efficacy of Watsu therapy in promoting rehabilitation and healing.

These narratives provide compelling evidence of the transformative impact of Watsu on individuals' physical and emotional well-being.

Collaborating with healthcare professionals: Collaboration with healthcare professionals is essential for incorporating Watsu therapy into comprehensive rehabilitation programs.

By collaborating with physicians, physical therapists, psychologists, and other healthcare providers, Watsu practitioners can ensure a multidisciplinary approach that addresses the diverse needs of patients.

CHAPTER 7
WATSU AND MENTAL WELLNESS

Water has long been associated with emotional healing and mental wellness, with various cultures recognizing its ability to promote relaxation and emotional balance. Watsu, a form of aquatic therapy developed in the 1980s by Harold Dull, takes advantage of these properties to offer a unique approach to healing and well-being. The understanding that water can facilitate

Connection Between Water and Emotional Healing:

Water has an innate ability to evoke feelings of calmness and tranquility in individuals. This connection between water and emotional healing stems from both psychological and physiological factors. Psychologically, water is often associated with purity, renewal, and serenity, which can have a profound impact on one's emotional state. Physiologically, being immersed in water triggers the release of endorphins, neurotransmitters that promote feelings of well-being and reduce stress and anxiety levels. In the context of Watsu therapy, the buoyancy and support provided by water create a safe and nurturing environment for emotional exploration and release. The gentle movements and stretches performed during a Watsu session encourage relaxation and help release tension held in the body, allowing clients to access and process buried emotions.

By combining physical touch with the soothing properties of water, Watsu facilitates a deep sense of connection and trust between the therapist and client, fostering emotional healing and growth.

<u>Using Watsu for Stress Reduction and Mental Clarity:</u>

Stress has become a pervasive issue in modern society, affecting individuals of all ages and backgrounds. Chronic stress not only takes a toll on physical health but also impacts mental well-being, contributing to anxiety, depression, and other mood disorders. Watsu offers a holistic approach to stress reduction, addressing both the physical and emotional aspects of stress. During a Watsu session, the rhythmic movements and gentle pressure applied by the therapist help release muscular tension and promote relaxation. The weightlessness experienced in the water relieves pressure on the joints and spine, allowing for greater freedom of movement and improved circulation.

Additionally, the sensory experience of being in water can shift focus away from stressful thoughts and promote a state of mental clarity and   presence. Combining Watsu with Mindfulness and Meditation   Techniques: Mindfulness and meditation are practices that involve cultivating awareness and presence in the present moment.

When combined with Watsu therapy, these practices can enhance the therapeutic benefits of both modalities. Mindfulness techniques, such as focused breathing and body scanning, can help clients deepen their connection to the sensations experienced during a Watsu session, allowing for greater relaxation and

emotional   release.
Meditation techniques, such as visualization
and guided imagery, can be incorporated into
Watsu sessions to promote mental well-being
and personal growth. For example, a therapist
may guide a client through a visualization
exercise while gently floating in the water,
encouraging them to imagine themselves
surrounded by healing light or immersed in a
peaceful natural setting.

These techniques can help clients tap into
their inner resources for healing and
resilience, empowering them to navigate life's
challenges with greater ease and clarity.
Watsu therapy offers a powerful tool for
promoting mental wellness and emotional
healing. By harnessing the therapeutic
properties of water and combining them with
mindfulness and meditation techniques,

Watsu provides a holistic approach to addressing stress, anxiety, and other emotional issues. Whether used as a standalone treatment or integrated into a comprehensive wellness plan, Watsu has the potential to transform lives and promote profound healing on a physical, emotional, and spiritual level.

CHAPTER 8
EXPANDING YOUR WATSU PRACTICE

Expanding a Watsu practice involves a multifaceted approach that encompasses various aspects ranging from client acquisition to professional development. To begin with, practitioners need to cultivate a deep understanding of the principles and techniques underlying Watsu aquatic therapy. This involves mastering the fundamentals of bodywork in water, including principles of buoyancy, support, and gentle movement. As practitioners become proficient in these foundational skills, they can begin to explore more advanced techniques such as stretches, joint mobilizations, and customized sessions tailored to individual client needs.

Moreover, expanding a Watsu practice necessitates a comprehensive understanding of client management and communication. Practitioners must be adept at conducting thorough assessments to identify client goals, preferences, and any contraindications or precautions. Clear and effective communication is essential throughout the therapeutic process to ensure client comfort, safety, and satisfaction. This may involve explaining the rationale behind specific techniques, addressing client concerns or questions, and soliciting feedback to inform treatment adjustments.

In addition to refining technical skills and communication abilities, expanding a Watsu practice requires strategic business development initiatives. This includes establishing efficient administrative processes, such as appointment scheduling, billing, and documentation, to streamline operations and enhance client experience. Moreover, practitioners need to cultivate a strong online presence through professional websites, social media platforms, and online directories to increase visibility and attract potential clients. Furthermore, building a robust referral network with other healthcare professionals, such as physicians, physical therapists, and chiropractors, can facilitate client referrals and enhance collaborative care opportunities. Networking within the broader wellness community through participation in conferences, workshops, and professional associations can also provide valuable exposure and networking opportunities. Ultimately, expanding a Watsu practice is an ongoing process that requires dedication, continuous learning, and adaptability.

By continually refining technical skills, enhancing communication abilities, and implementing strategic business development initiatives, practitioners can effectively grow their client base, increase their impact, and contribute to the broader advancement of aquatic therapy.

Building a Clientele and Marketing Your Services:

Building a clientele and effectively marketing Watsu services requires a strategic approach that combines targeted outreach, compelling messaging, and personalized engagement. Central to this endeavor is cultivating a deep understanding of the target demographic and their unique needs, preferences, and challenges.

This involves conducting market research to identify potential client segments, including individuals seeking relief from chronic pain, stress management, rehabilitation from injuries or surgeries, and holistic wellness enthusiasts.

Once the target audience has been identified, practitioners can tailor their marketing efforts to resonate with their specific needs and interests. This may involve crafting compelling messaging that highlights the benefits of Watsu therapy in addressing common concerns such as pain relief, relaxation, improved mobility, and enhanced overall well-being. Utilizing a variety of marketing channels, including social media, email newsletters, print materials, and word-of-mouth referrals, can help reach and engage prospective clients across diverse demographics and platforms. In addition to traditional marketing tactics, practitioners can leverage digital platforms and technology to expand their reach and enhance client engagement. Developing a professional website that showcases the practice's services, credentials, testimonials, and educational resources can serve as a valuable tool for attracting and informing potential clients. Incorporating search engine optimization (SEO) strategies to improve online visibility and utilizing online scheduling and payment systems can further streamline the client acquisition process and enhance convenience.

Moreover, building a clientele requires cultivating strong relationships and fostering trust with prospective clients. This involves actively listening to their concerns, addressing any questions or apprehensions they may have, and providing personalized recommendations or treatment plans tailored to their individual needs and goals.

Offering introductory sessions, promotional discounts, or referral incentives can incentivize prospective clients to try Watsu therapy and help build a loyal client base over time.

Continuing Education and Advanced Training Opportunities: Continuing education and advanced training are essential components of professional development for Watsu practitioners seeking to deepen their knowledge, refine their skills, and stay abreast of emerging trends and innovations in aquatic therapy. As the field of Watsu therapy continues to evolve, practitioners must remain committed to lifelong learning and ongoing skill development to provide the highest quality of care to their clients. One avenue for continuing education is participation in advanced training programs and workshops offered by reputable organizations and experienced instructors. These programs may cover specialized topics such as advanced techniques in aquatic bodywork, specialized populations (e.g., Pediatrics, geriatrics, athletes), therapeutic interventions for specific conditions (e.g., chronic pain, neurological disorders, post-surgical rehabilitation), and integrative approaches combining Watsu with other complementary modalities. Moreover, pursuing advanced certifications and credentials can enhance professional credibility, expand scope of practice, and differentiate practitioners in the marketplace. Certifying bodies such as the Worldwide Aquatic Bodywork Association (WABA) and the Aquatic Therapy & Rehab Institute (ATRI) offer specialized certifications and credentialing pathways for Watsu practitioners seeking to demonstrate proficiency in advanced techniques and specialized areas of practice. Additionally, staying abreast of current research and literature in the field of aquatic therapy through academic journals, conferences, and online resources can provide valuable insights into best practices, evidence-based interventions, and emerging trends. Engaging in peer-to-peer networking and mentorship opportunities within the Watsu community can also facilitate knowledge sharing, collaboration, and professional growth.

Establishing Watsu Communities and Networks:

Establishing Watsu communities and networks plays a vital role in fostering collaboration, camaraderie, and professional support among practitioners, instructors, and enthusiasts within the field of aquatic therapy. By coming together to share knowledge, experiences, and resources, Watsu communities can promote continuous learning, innovation, and advancement in the practice of aquatic therapy. One way to establish Watsu communities is through the formation of local or regional practitioner groups or chapters affiliated with larger professional organizations such as the Worldwide Aquatic Bodywork Association (WABA) or the Aquatic Therapy & Rehab

Institute (ATRI). These groups can facilitate regular meetings, workshops, and peer-to-peer mentoring opportunities to exchange ideas, discuss challenging cases, and provide mutual support.

Moreover, leveraging digital platforms and social media channels can help connect Watsu practitioners across geographic boundaries and facilitate virtual networking and knowledge sharing. Online forums, discussion groups, and social media communities dedicated to aquatic therapy can serve as valuable resources for practitioners to seek advice, share insights, and stay connected with peers and mentors. Furthermore, organizing and participating in community outreach initiatives, such as wellness fairs, health expos, and educational workshops, can help raise awareness about the benefits of Watsu therapy and expand access to aquatic therapy services within the broader community. Collaborating with local healthcare providers, wellness centers, and recreational facilities can also create opportunities for interdisciplinary collaboration and referral networking. Overall, establishing Watsu communities and networks is essential for nurturing a supportive and collaborative ecosystem that empowers practitioners to thrive personally and professionally. By fostering a culture of inclusivity, collaboration, and continuous learning, Watsu communities can contribute to the advancement and sustainability of aquatic therapy as a valuable modality for promoting health, healing, and well-being.

CHAPTER 9
EXPLORING THE FUTURE OF WATSU

The exploration of the future of Watsu, a form of aquatic therapy, encompasses a multifaceted examination of potential advancements, adaptations, and expansions within the field. As society continues to evolve, so too does the landscape of healthcare and wellness practices. Watsu, which combines elements of water-based therapy, massage, and meditation, holds promise for continued development and innovation. One avenue for exploration lies in the integration of emerging technologies into Watsu practices. This could involve the development of specialized equipment or digital tools aimed at enhancing the therapeutic experience for both practitioners and clients.

For instance, advancements in hydrotherapy pools or wearable devices designed to monitor physiological responses during Watsu sessions could revolutionize the way in which therapy is administered and assessed.

Moreover, the future of Watsu may also involve a deeper understanding of its potential applications across diverse populations and settings. Research into the efficacy of Watsu for specific conditions or demographics, such as pediatric patients or individuals with disabilities, could inform tailored approaches to treatment. Additionally, the incorporation of complementary practices, such as mindfulness techniques or aromatherapy, may further expand the scope and impact of Watsu therapy.

Ultimately, the future of Watsu holds promise for continued innovation, growth, and integration within the broader landscape of holistic healthcare. Innovations in Aquatic Therapy Technology: Innovations in aquatic therapy technology represent a significant area of interest and potential advancement within the field of Watsu. As technology continues to progress, opportunities emerge to enhance the delivery, effectiveness, and accessibility of aquatic therapy interventions. One area of innovation involves the development of specialized equipment designed specifically for use in water-based therapy sessions. This could include ergonomic flotation devices, adjustable massage tables, or underwater exercise equipment tailored to the unique needs of therapists and clients. Furthermore, advancements in hydrotherapy pool design and maintenance may also contribute to improved outcomes and experiences for individuals participating in aquatic therapy programs. For example, the integration of temperature control systems, water filtration technologies, and customizable features could optimize the therapeutic environment and ensure maximum comfort and safety for all participants. Additionally, the use of digital technologies holds promise for enhancing the monitoring and assessment of therapy sessions. Wearable devices capable of tracking movement, heart rate, and other physiological metrics can provide valuable data insights to therapists and inform personalized treatment plans. Moreover, the development of virtual reality or augmented reality platforms may offer immersive therapeutic experiences that complement traditional aquatic therapy techniques. By embracing innovations in technology, the field of aquatic therapy stands poised to evolve and expand its reach, ultimately improving outcomes for individuals seeking rehabilitation, pain management, or holistic wellness. Research and Evidence-Based Practices in Watsu:

Research and evidence-based practices play a crucial role in advancing the field of Watsu and validating its efficacy as a therapeutic modality. While Watsu has gained recognition for its potential benefits in promoting relaxation, pain relief, and emotional well-being, further empirical research is needed to substantiate these claims and refine treatment protocols.

One avenue for research involves conducting controlled clinical trials to evaluate the effectiveness of Watsu for specific medical conditions or populations.

By comparing outcomes between Watsu interventions and standard care or alternative therapies, researchers can elucidate the relative benefits and limitations of aquatic therapy in various contexts. Additionally, qualitative studies exploring the lived experiences of individuals undergoing Watsu treatment can provide valuable insights into its subjective effects and mechanisms of action. Furthermore, research into the physiological and neurobiological effects of Watsu may shed light on its underlying mechanisms and inform evidence-based practice guidelines. For instance, studies examining changes in heart rate variability, stress hormone levels, or neural activity during Watsu sessions can contribute to our understanding of how water-based therapy impacts the body and mind.

Moreover, collaborative efforts between researchers, therapists, and healthcare providers are essential for translating research findings into clinical practice and integrating Watsu into mainstream healthcare systems.

By fostering a culture of inquiry and evidence-based decision-making, the field of Watsu can continue to evolve and thrive as a legitimate therapeutic approach for promoting holistic wellness and healing. Global Trends and Opportunities in Watsu

Therapy:

The global landscape of Watsu therapy is shaped by a myriad of trends and opportunities that reflect the evolving needs, preferences, and challenges facing individuals and communities worldwide. One prominent trend is the growing recognition and acceptance of complementary and alternative therapies within mainstream healthcare systems. As interest in holistic approaches to health and wellness continues to rise, opportunities emerge for Watsu therapists to collaborate with conventional medical practitioners and expand their reach to new patient populations. Additionally, demographic shifts and societal changes, such as aging populations and increasing stress levels, create demand for therapeutic interventions that address both physical and psychological well-being.

Watsu therapy, with its emphasis on gentle movement, mindfulness, and the healing properties of water, is uniquely positioned to meet these evolving needs and preferences. Furthermore, globalization and advances in communication technology have facilitated the exchange of knowledge and expertise across geographic boundaries, opening up opportunities for cross-cultural collaboration and innovation within the field of Watsu.

By embracing multicultural perspectives and adapting practices to suit diverse cultural contexts, Watsu therapists can enhance the accessibility and relevance of their services on a global scale. Moreover, the proliferation of wellness tourism and the emergence of specialized retreats and resorts focused on holistic healing experiences present opportunities for Watsu practitioners to showcase their skills and attract clientele from around the world. By staying attuned to global trends and seizing opportunities for innovation and collaboration, Watsu therapy can continue to thrive as a valuable component of the international wellness landscape, offering healing and rejuvenation to individuals across cultures and continents.

CONCLUSION

Watsu aquatic therapy represents a dynamic and evolving field with vast potential for growth, innovation, and impact on holistic health and well-being. From exploring the future of Watsu to embracing innovations in aquatic therapy technology, conducting research to validate evidence-based practices, and capitalizing on global trends and opportunities, there are numerous avenues for advancing the field and maximizing its benefits for individuals and communities worldwide. By fostering interdisciplinary collaboration, integrating emerging technologies, and staying abreast of evolving healthcare trends, Watsu therapists can continue to refine their skills, expand their reach, and contribute to the advancement of aquatic therapy as a recognized and respected modality within mainstream healthcare systems. Ultimately, the principles of Watsu — fostering connection, promoting relaxation, and harnessing the healing power of water — have the potential to inspire profound transformations in mind, body, and spirit, offering hope, healing, and renewal to all who

seek its therapeutic embrace.